WILDERNESS SELF RELIANCE

Survival situations are inherently hazardous. You are likely lost or incapacitated, exhausted, sleep deprived, hungry and stressed. That makes a perfect formula for the added injury of a fall or misstep resulting in a sprain, or a gash or cut from a wayward branch. Or you may have eaten or drank something that has caused stomach upset resulting in gastric distress and dehydration. If you are surviving in extreme temperature, you are facing the added need to protect your core body temperature so your brain and body can function properly.

While this guide focuses on medicinal plants that are found in the eastern woodlands of the United States, these plants are likely to be found in other settings as well. Learning these may help you survive, no matter where you are.

The Pathfinder School System®

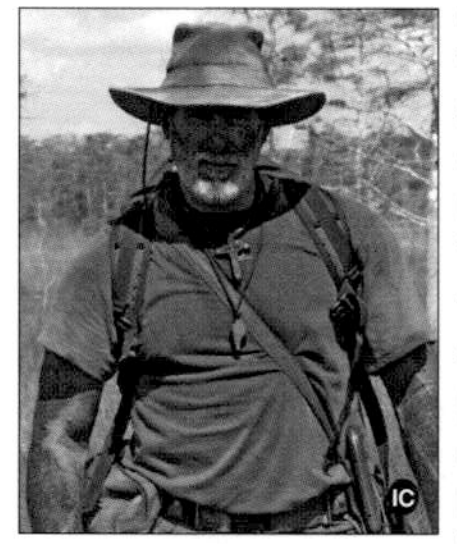

Created as a teaching tool for my students in Wilderness Self Reliance, the Pathfinder School System represents the wisdom of the ancient scouts who ventured ahead of nomadic tribes to find fresh areas to support their community.

These "Pathfinders" had to accurately identify the perfect spot to sustain their tribes – they had to recognize the resources that would afford food, shelter, water, medicine and protection – the very same resources a person would need today.

What to Know

- Where it is an option, your first choice is to seek medical attention from a qualified medical professional. If that is not possible, you should be prepared to recognize what conditions are likely to occur, what plants and other medicinal resources are available, and to know how to use them for specific purposes.
- While there are numerous medicinal species, commit 8 to 10 species to memory that you can identify in all seasons in their preferred habitats. Practice identifying species at botanic gardens and garden shops before you need this knowledge.

Dave Canterbury is a master woodsman with over 20 years of experience working in many dangerous environments. He has taught outdoor survival around the world, and his common sense approach to survivability is recognized as one of the most effective systems of teaching known today. For information on Pathfinder programs and materials visit:

www.thepathfinderschoolllc.com

Measurements refer to the height of plants unless otherwiswe indicated. The species are coded according to seasonal availability:

Spring Summer Autumn Winter

N.B. – The publisher makes no representation or warranties with respect to the accuracy, completeness, correctness or usefulness of this information and specifically disclaims any implied warranties of fitness for a particular purpose. The advice, strategies and/or techniques contained herein may not be suitable for all individuals. The publisher shall not be responsible for any physical harm (up to and including death), loss of profit or other commercial damage. The publisher assumes no liability brought or instituted by individuals or organizations arising out of or relating in any way to the application and/or use of the information, advice and strategies contained herein. Laminated, water resistant, do not submerge.

Waterford Press publishes reference guides that introduce readers to nature observation, outdoor recreation and survival skills. Product information is featured on the website: **www.waterfordpress.com.**

$7.95 U.S.
$9.95 CAN

ISBN 978-1-58355-708-2

Text & illustrations © 2014, 2023 Waterford Press Inc. All rights reserved. Images marked IC © Iris Canterbury 2014, 2023.

To order or for information on custom published products please call 800-434-2555 or email orderdesk@waterfordpress.com. For permissions or to share comments email editor@waterfordpress.com. 2300604

10 9 8 7 6 5 4 3 2 1

Made in the USA

MEDICINAL PLANTS OF THE EASTERN WOODLANDS – A Waterproof Folding Guide to Familiar Species

PATHFINDER OUTDOOR SURVIVAL GUIDE™

MEDICINAL PLANTS OF THE EASTERN WOODLANDS

A Waterproof Folding Guide to Familiar Species

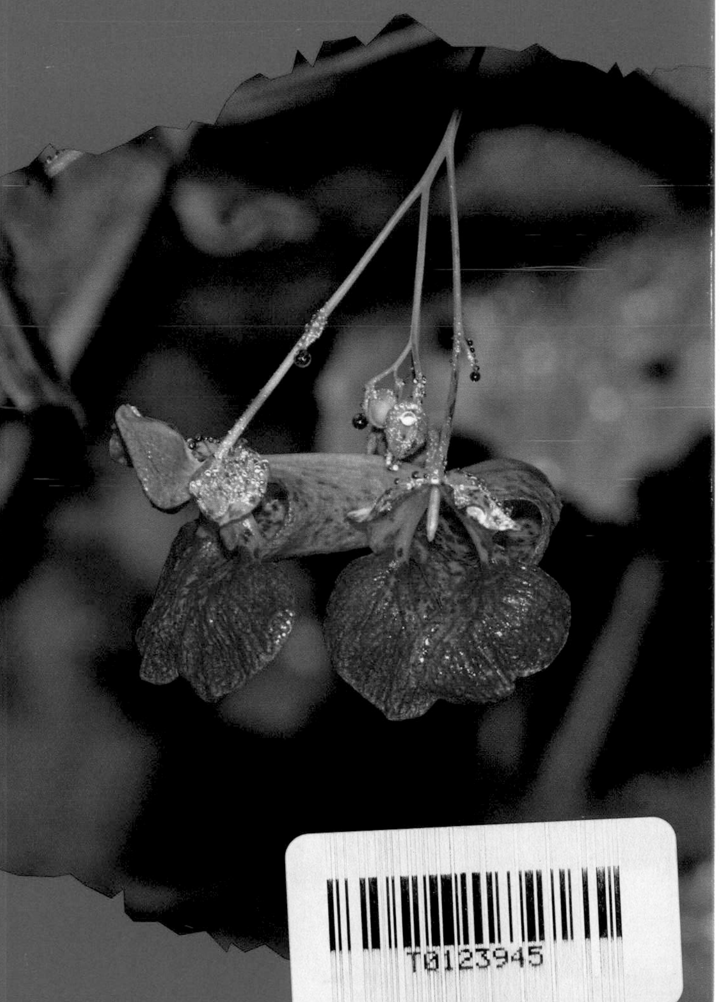

THE PATHFINDER SCHOOL

www.thepathfinderschoolllc.com

WHEN TO USE MEDICINAL PLANTS

Conditions That Warrant Survival Treatment

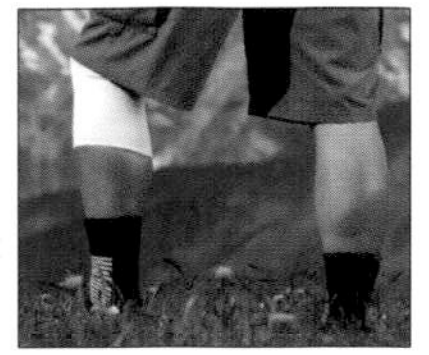

In a survival situation, avoid making your situation worse by not treating injuries or illness that can further incapacitate you over time. In addition to basic first aid training and the strategies outlined in our Wilderness First Aid guide, you can use medicinal plants to help treat and relieve injuries/conditions and avoid infections.

Cuts Present a Risk of Infection and Blood Loss – Use plants with antiseptic qualities like raspberry, yarrow and goldenrod to clean the wound. If bleeding is severe, use a poultice of plantain or yarrow leaves to help blood coagulate.

Open Wounds/Sores – Infection is nearly inevitable in a survival situation. Signs of an infected wound include increasing pain, redness and swelling, white pus, red streaks under the skin near the wound and fever. Continue to clean and dress the wound several times a day until the infection subsides.

Rashes/Fungal Infections – Chaffing and fungal infections, especially to your legs and feet, will impair your ability to walk. Use plants that have antiseptic qualities to clean wounds. Cushion distressed areas and avoid further irritation by using mosses if available. Treat rashes as open wounds and dress them daily until healed.

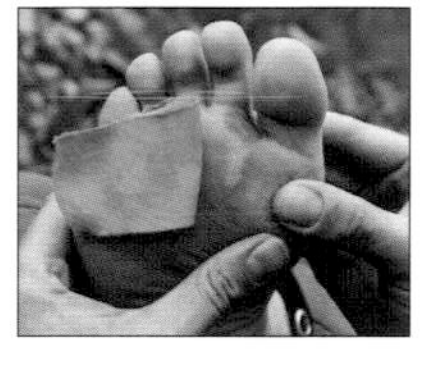

For dry weeping rashes, make a compress of vinegar or tannic acid from a tea of boiled acorns or the bark of a hardwood tree. Sphagnum moss, found in boggy areas worldwide, is a natural source of iodine. Use as a dressing.

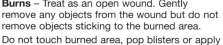

Burns – Treat as an open wound. Gently remove any objects from the wound but do not remove objects sticking to the burned area.

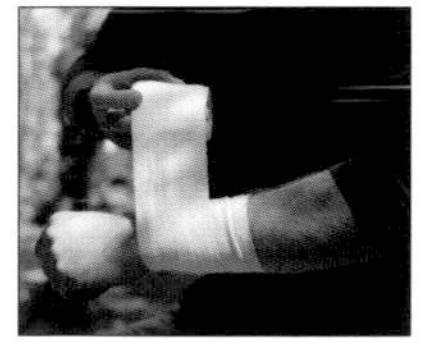

Do not touch burned area, pop blisters or apply ointments. Relieve pain by pouring cold water over the area until pain subsides. Make decoction of oak tree bark or acorns, soak sterile dressings in this and cover the wound gently to prevent infection.

Contact Dermatitis – Some plants exude an oil that causes extreme skin irritation. Symptoms include burning, reddening, itching, swelling and blistering and may take hours or even days to appear. The effects are spread by scratching and the oil can also get on gear which will infect whoever touches it. When symptoms first appear, it is recommended to wash the affected area with water repeatedly. If water is not readily available, use dirt or sand. Once the oil has been removed, itching can be relieved by crushing jewelweed plants and rubbing the juice on the skin.

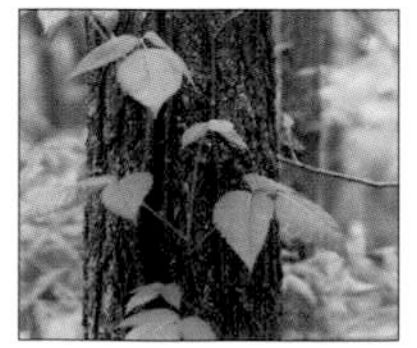

A Little Common Sense®

- NEVER taste or use any wild plant in a medical procedure unless you are CERTAIN of its identification.
- ALWAYS properly prepare plants for their intended use.

PREPARING MEDICINAL PLANTS

Infusion or Tea – An infusion is a process that allows botanical chemicals to be extracted from plants. Generally, an infusion made from roots or bark should be left to steep longer than those made from flowers or leaves. Fresh plants tend to infuse much faster than dried plants. The length of time the "tea" steeps also affects the strength of the infusion.

- ***Hot Infusion Preparation:***
  1. Pour boiling water over 1 oz.* of freshly shredded plant material.
  2. Cover the brew.
  3. Let it steep for 5-15 minutes.
  4. After steeping, filter out the plant matter and use the liquid.
- ***Cold Infusion Preparation:***
  1. Same as above using cold water.

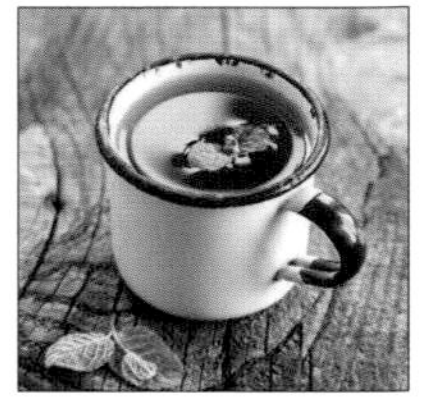

Expressed Juice – Liquids or saps squeezed from plants and applied directly on wounds or used to create other medicines.

Decoction – This process extracts chemicals from plants by boiling them for an extended period. Decoctions are usually made of harder plant materials including bark, stems, roots and nutshells.

- ***Preparation:***
  1. Pour a cup of water into a container and bring to a boil.
  2. Add 1-2 oz.* of plant parts to the water; continue simmering over low heat for 15-30 minutes.
  3. Remove from heat and let the brew stand for a few minutes.
  4. Strain the liquid out while it is still hot.

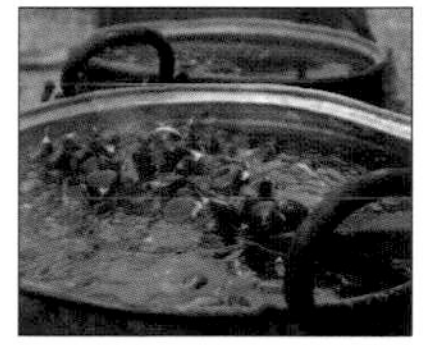

Poultices, Fomentations and Compresses

Poultices, fomentations and compresses are used to draw out infections (and splinters) and are applied directly to the skin. Herbal poultices and fomentation should be kept in place for 1-24 hours as needed. During this period you may experience a throbbing pain as it draws out the infection and neutralizes toxins. You will know that the treatment is working when the pain subsides, at which point the dressing should be removed.

Poultice – Ground, masticated (chewed), or shredded herbs are packed over the skin and then wrapped to keep in place.

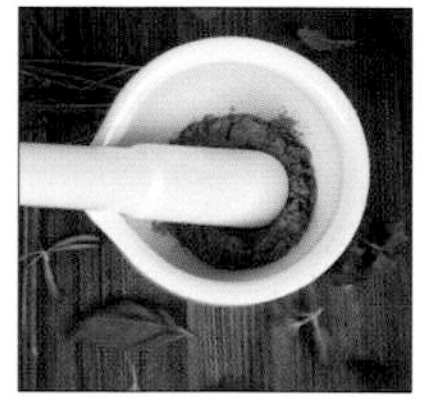

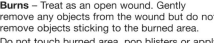

Poultices are made by crushing plant parts.

Hot Poultice – Best for superficial wounds; the heat helps to draw blood to the surface, opens the pores, and assists in the assimilation of the herbs through the skin. Great for wet and unproductive coughs.

- ***Preparation:***
  1. If using fresh herbs for your poultice, place 4 oz. of bruised or chopped herbs and 1 cup of water in a pot. Warm for 2 minutes. Do not drain.
  2. Arrange a clean piece of cloth on a clean, flat surface. Place the hot herbs on the skin you are treating. The material should be large enough to cover the affected area completely. Pour the liquid herbal solution over the cloth and place the cloth over the herbs that are on the skin. Wrap a towel around the poultice to contain the solution.

*NOTE: A large egg weighs about two ounces.

PREPARING MEDICINAL PLANTS

Cold Poultice – Best for deep wounds such as contusions, bruises, fractures, etc; the affected area will usually feel "hot" to touch and so the cold poultice (made either by preparing herbs with cold water or by cooling a previously prepared one) will act as an analgesic – helping to draw the effects of the herbs down deep into the tissue.

- ***Preparation:***
  1. Same as above using cold water.

Spit Poultice (Compress) – An instant poultice made by chewing plants and applying to affected area.

Fomentation – Dip a cloth or towel into a warm infusion or decoction, wring it out and put on the affected body part. Cover the cloth with a dry towel to help retain the heat. These herbal preparations are used to treat headaches, chest congestion, skin irritations, and swelling due to an injury. They can be used hot or cold. On open wounds, use cold compresses. Use hot compresses when the skin is not broken and/or circulation needs to be brought to the area.

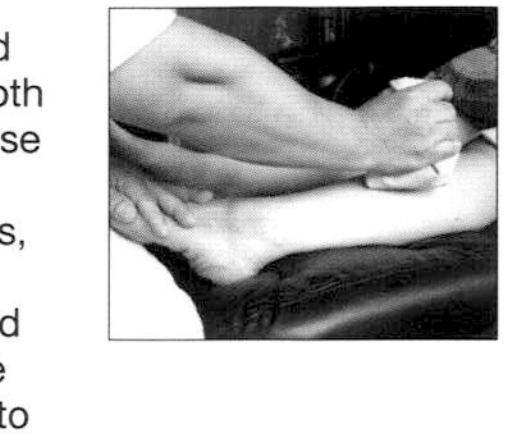

History & Medicinal Plants

Healing what ails us with plants has been around as long as the history of man. The works of Hippocrates himself contains over 300 medicinal plants, such as garlic, wormwood and nightshade. Marco Polo's visits to Asia, China and Persia resulted in many medicinal plants being brought to Europe. Native Americans have used herbs and plants to heal the body for thousands of years.

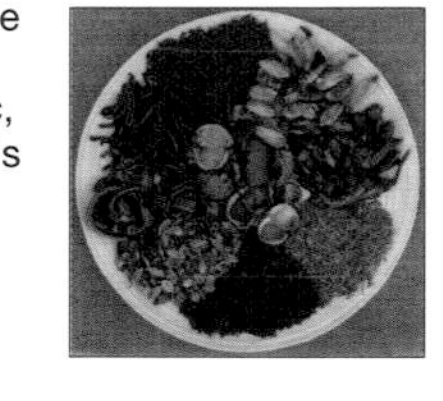

EASTERN WOODLANDS

The eastern woodlands is a region that encompasses three distinct forest types:

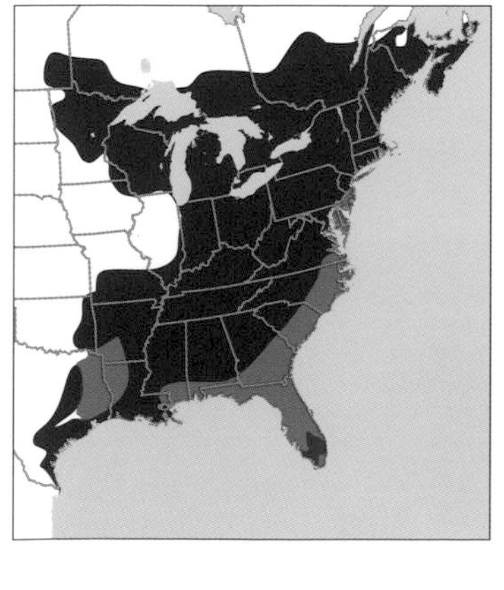

Temperate, Broadleaf & Mixed Forest
Forest biome is dominated by deciduous trees that lose their leaves in autumn. Dominant species include oaks, maples, hickories, beeches and elms.

Temperate Coniferous Forest
A mixed forest of conifers, evergreen broadleaf trees and deciduous broadleafs.

Flooded Grassland & Savanna
Dominant species include mangroves, cypresses, pines, palms, gum trees and figs.

SAFETY FIRST

The most important consideration when foraging for medicinal plants is to avoid poisoning from toxic plants. Some, like poison ivy, poison oak and giant hogweed, are toxic when contacted and can cause skin rashes and blistering. Never burn them for fuel since the smoke is also toxic.

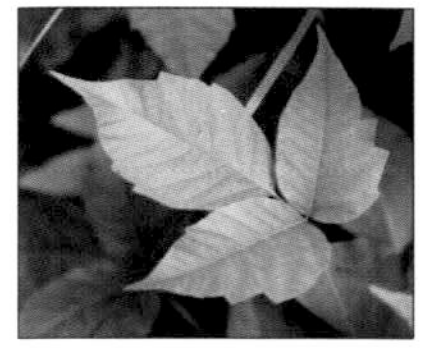

Poison Ivy
Small shrub or trailing vine has leaves with 3 leaflets.

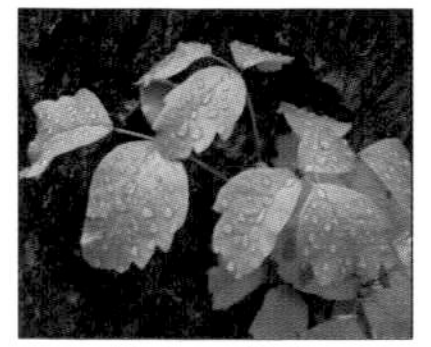

Poison Oak
Small shrub or trailing vine. Oak-like leaves have 3 leaflets.

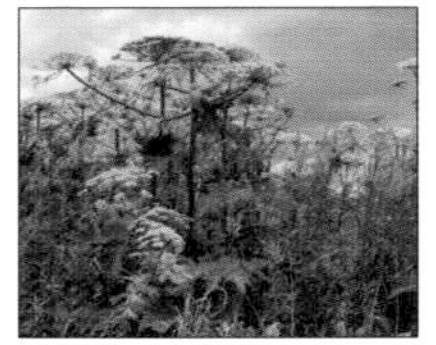

Giant Hogweed
Huge plant up to 23 ft. (7 m) tall has flat-topped clusters of white flowers.

- Never collect plants growing in contaminated water or from water that might contain parasites (like giardia). If you need to use questionable plants, boil them in water for 15 minutes and discard the water.
- Signs of potentially poisonous plants include:
  - Milky sap
  - Seeds or beans inside pods
  - Bitter or soapy taste
  - Grains with pink to blackish spurs
  - Spines, thorns or fine hairs
  - Parsley or carrot-like foliage
  - Almond-scented
  - Leaves grow in "threes"
- Make sure you have positively identified the species and that it is right for the condition you are attempting to remedy.

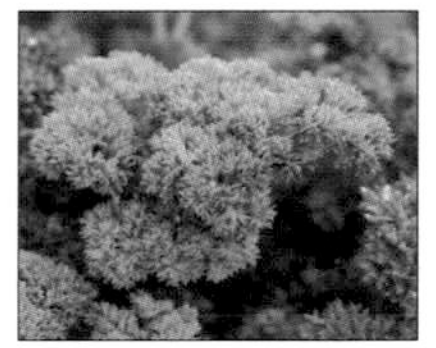

Parsley-like foliage

PLANT PARTS

SIMPLE LEAF SHAPES

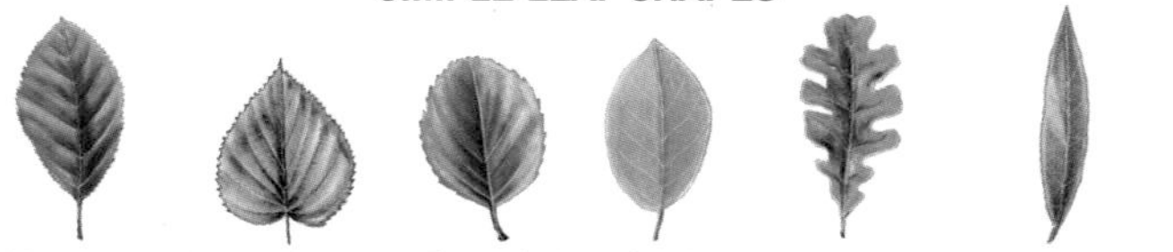

Elliptical, Heart-shaped, Rounded, Oval, Lobed, Lance-shaped

COMPOUND LEAVES

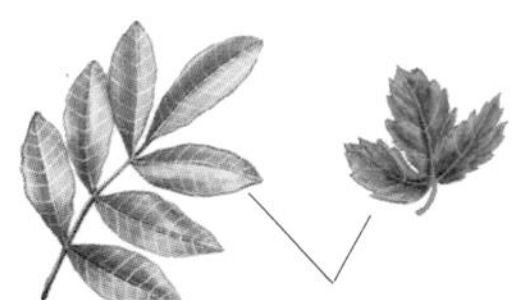

Leaflets

LEAF ARRANGEMENTS

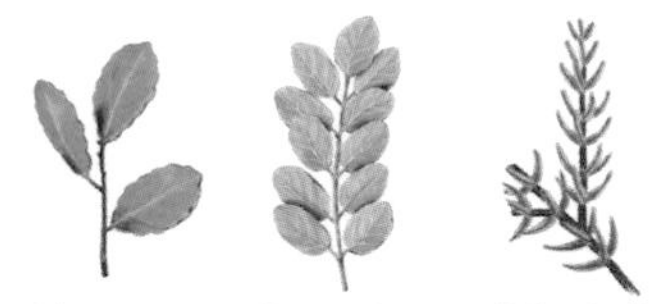

Alternate, Opposite, Whorled

FLOWER SHAPES

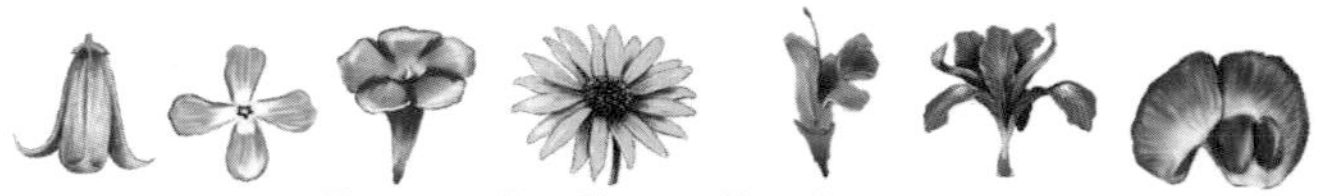

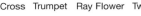

Bell, Cross, Trumpet, Ray Flower, Two-lipped, Iris, Pea-shaped

TREES & SHRUBS

TREES & SHRUBS

WILDFLOWERS

WILDFLOWERS

WILDFLOWERS

PLANTS SORTED BY AILMENT

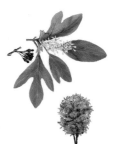

Sassafras
Sassafras albidum
To 100 ft. (18 m)

Description: Shrub or small tree has a crown of short, thick branches. Opposite leaves are simple or lobed and often mitten-shaped. Yellowish flowers bloom in a cluster at the end of twig tips and are succeeded by blue-black, single-seeded fruits.
Habitat: Moist, sandy soils, mixed woodlands, valleys.
Harvest: Roots.
Uses: Diuretic, emetic, tonic. Tea was once believed a cure-all that could successfully treat conditions including fatigue, stomachaches, colds, fevers, gout, high blood pressure, kidney ailments, rheumatism, chest, bowel and liver disorders and can be used as a wash for skin irritations and ulcers.
Comments: Use sparingly. The oil found in sassafras is reportedly carcinogenic and is banned by the FDA.

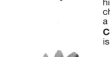
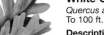
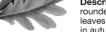

White Oak
Quercus alba
To 100 ft. (30 m)

Description: Large, stout-trunked tree has a large, rounded crown of spreading branches. Lobed leaves are widest above the middle, turn red-brown in autumn and often stay attached to the tree throughout the winter.
Habitat: Moist, well-drained soils, dry woods, often in pure stands.
Harvest: Bark, leaves.
Uses: Astringent, antiseptic, tonic. Inner bark tea was **drank** to treat diarrhea, excessive mucous discharge, bleeding and piles, **gargled** to treat throat infections and **applied externally** as a wash for poison ivy rash, burns and to stop bleeding.
Comments: Tannic acid in bark has anti-tumor properties and has been used to treat cancers and inflammatory skin diseases.

Yellowroot
Xanthorhiza simplicissima
To 3 ft. (90 cm)

Description: Small shrub has erect, unbranched stems. Leaves are divided into 5-toothed leaflets. Small brown-purple flowers bloom in spring. Root is deep yellow.
Habitat: Moist woodlands, streambanks, thickets.
Harvest: Root.
Uses: Anti-inflammatory, astringent. Root tea is used to alleviate colds, cramps, sore throat or mouth, and hypertension. Poultice is applied externally for piles.
Comments: Is potentially toxic in large doses.

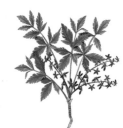
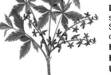

Tulip Poplar
Liriodendron tulipifera
To 120 ft. (36.5 m)

Description: Tall tree has a straight trunk and brown, furrowed bark. Leaves have evenly rounded lobes. Tulip-like, greenish to yellow-orange flowers have 6 petals. Fruit is a reddish cone-shaped structure composed of pointed fruits.
Habitat: Moist soils in mixed forests
Harvest: Leaves, bark.
Uses: Bark tea is a cure-all for indigestion, rheumatism, fevers, coughs, toothaches and malaria. It can be used externally as a wash for wounds and bites. A poultice of leaves helps relieve headaches.
Comments: One of the first trees to turn yellow and lose its leaves in autumn.

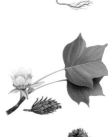
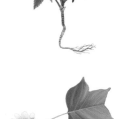
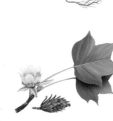
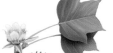
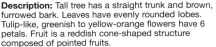
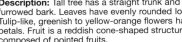

Pitch Pine
Pinus rigida
To 6 ft. (30 m)

Description: Medium-sized tree often has an irregular crown of horizontal branches. Needles are bundled in 3s and tufts of needles often grow on the trunk. Fruit is a woody, egg-shaped cone.
Habitat: Sandy, rocky and acidic soils, steep slopes to river valleys.
Harvest: Needles, sap (pitch).
Uses: Irritant, antiseptic, diuretic. Apply pitch to relieve joint inflammation and help open sores to heal. Rub pitch on splinters and they will pop out within 48 hours. Needle tea is an excellent source of vitamin C.
Comments: This is the dominant species of the New Jersey pine barrens.

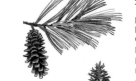

White Pine
Pinus strobus
To 100 ft. (30 m)

Description: Tree has straight trunk and crown of horizontal branches. Needles are bundled in 5s. Cylindrical cones are long-stalked.
Habitat: Well-drained soils in a variety of habitats.
Harvest: Needles, bark, sap.
Uses: Tea of needles and inner bark alleviates coughs, colds and sore throats and is an excellent source of vitamin C. Poultices of leaves and bark are used to treat headaches and backaches. Sap is applied to help wounds heal, draw out infections, ease joint pain and reduce inflammation.
Comments: Also known as the eastern white pine, northern white pine and soft pine.

Black Walnut
Juglans nigra
To 150 ft. (46 m)

Description: Alternate leaves have 9-21 leaflets. Opposite, lance-shaped, wrinkled leaves are joined across the stem at their bases. Small, dull-white flowers bloom in dense, flat-topped clusters.
Habitat: Mixed deciduous forests, bottomlands.
Harvest: Bark, husks, leaves.
Uses: Anti-inflammatory, antiseptic, anti-fungal. Infusion of inner bark or buds treats colds, constipation and is an appetite stimulant and tonic. Leaf tea is used to prevent infection and is also an insecticide. Bark can be chewed for toothache.
Comments: Many believe walnut derivatives target parasites and can be used to treat cancer.

Black Willow
Salix nigra
To 100 ft. (30 m)

Description: Tree usually has more than one trunk. Alternate leaves are narrow, lance-shaped and finely saw-toothed. Bark is blackish. Flowers bloom in long catkins and are succeeded by reddish seed capsules.
Habitat: Wet areas, floodplains, streambanks.
Harvest: Leaves, bark.
Uses: Astringent, anti-inflammatory, tonic, diuretic. Poulticed leaves help wounds to heal. Decoction of tree bark is used to relieve headaches, fever and diarrhea. Decoction is also a good wash for wounds.
Comments: Other common names include noseblead plant, milfoil, soldier's woundwort and devil's nettle.

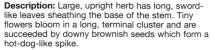

Dwarf Cinquefoil
Potentilla canadensis
To 6 in. (15 cm)

Description: Low-growing plant with hairy, reddish stems spreads like a vine. Leaves have 5 leaflets toothed above the middle. Yellow, 5-petaled flowers bloom at stem tips.
Habitat: Dry, open areas, fields, open woods.
Harvest: Roots, leaves.
Uses: Astringent, tonic. Tea of pounded roots relieves diarrhea.
Comments: Also called five-finger cinquefoil.

Cattail
Typha latifolia
To 10 ft. (3 m)

Description: Large, upright herb has long, sword-like leaves sheathing the base of the stem. Tiny flowers bloom in a long, terminal cluster and are succeeded by downy brownish seeds which form a hot-dog-like spike.
Habitat: Shallow margins of lakes, ponds, marshes, ditches.
Harvest: Roots, shoots.
Uses: The gel at the base of cattail roots is an antiseptic and provides relief from burns and stings. A poultice of roots helps wounds and burns to heal. Use young shoots as toothbrushes.
Comments: The leaves can also be burned to create an antiseptic that stops bleeding.

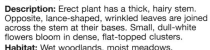
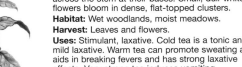
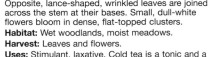
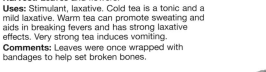
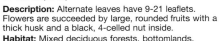

Boneset
Eupatorium perfoliatum
To 4 ft. (1.2 m)

Description: Erect plant has a thick, hairy stem. Opposite, lance-shaped, wrinkled leaves are joined across the stem at their bases. Small, dull-white flowers bloom in dense, flat-topped clusters.
Habitat: Wet woodlands, moist meadows.
Harvest: Leaves and flowers.
Uses: Stimulant, laxative. Cold tea is a tonic and a mild laxative. Warm tea can promote sweating and aids in breaking fevers and has strong laxative effects. Very strong tea induces vomiting.
Comments: Leaves were once wrapped with bandages to help set broken bones.

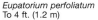

Yarrow
Achillea millefolium
To 40 in. (1 m)

Description: Creeping, erect plant has woolly stems and soft, feathery, fern-like leaves. Small white or pinkish flowers bloom in dense, flat-topped terminal clusters.
Habitat: Fields, grasslands, waste areas, roadsides.
Harvest: Entire plant.
Uses: Astringent, tonic, diuretic, stops bleeding. Hot tea opens up the pores, promotes sweating and can help break fevers. Cold teas acts as a digestive stimulant and diuretic. Crushed leaves will help blood to coagulate; a spit poultice stuffed in a nostril will stop a nosebleed.
Comments: Other common names include noseblead plant, milfoil, soldier's woundwort and devil's nettle.

Common Mullein
Verbascum thapsus
To 6 ft. (3 m)

Description: Common roadside weed has broad leaves covered in gray hairs. Yellow flowers bloom in a long terminal spike.
Habitat: Waste areas, roadsides, fields, poor soils.
Harvest: Flowers, leaves, stalks.
Uses: Tea of leaves or flowers can be used as an expectorant, decongestant, diuretic, cold and headache remedy. Absorbent, antibacterial leaves can be used as dressings in a variety of applications and as toilet paper.
Comments: Younger plants have more potent effects. The leaves have traditionally been smoked to relieve coughs, asthma and minor mental disorders.

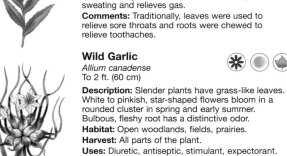

Goldenrod
Solidago spp.
To 7 ft. (2.1 m)

Description: Tall, erect plant has alternate, stalkless leaves. Small yellow flowers bloom in arching, terminal clusters.
Habitat: Dry open woods and fields, meadows, often on sandy soil.
Harvest: Leaves, flowers.
Uses: Astringent, diuretic, stimulant. Tea promotes sweating and relieves gas.
Comments: Traditionally, leaves were used to relieve sore throats and roots were chewed to relieve toothaches.

Wild Garlic
Allium canadense
To 2 ft. (60 cm)

Description: Slender plants have grass-like leaves. White to pinkish, star-shaped flowers bloom in a rounded cluster in spring and early summer. Bulbous, fleshy root has a distinctive odor.
Habitat: Open woodlands, fields, prairies.
Harvest: All parts of the plant.
Uses: Diuretic, antiseptic, stimulant, expectorant. Juice is used as antiseptic. Teas treat coughing, colds, flus, relieve stomach cramps and wind, promote sweating and improve blood circulation.
Comments: Despite its common name, the plant bulb tastes of onion.

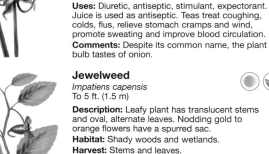
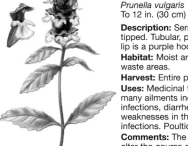
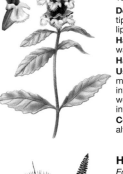
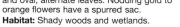

Jewelweed
Impatiens capensis
To 5 ft. (1.5 m)

Description: Leafy plant has translucent stems and oval, alternate leaves. Nodding gold to orange flowers have a spurred sac.
Habitat: Shady woods and wetlands.
Harvest: Stems and leaves.
Uses: Antiseptic, stops bleeding, promotes healing. Crush plant and apply juice to rashes and cuts. Provides relief from rashes caused by contact poison plants.
Comments: Often grows in the same habitats as poison ivy.

Plantain
Plantago major
To 18 in. (45 cm)

Description: Common weed. Basal leaves have wavy edges. Greenish flowers have purplish anthers and bloom in long spikes.
Habitat: Fields, ditches, wet meadows, disturbed areas.
Harvest: Entire plant.
Uses: Astringent, diuretic, expectorant. Has strong drawing properties; use a poultice to draw out poisons from stings or bites; will even draw out splinters and thorns. Apply poultice of leaves to cuts to stop bleeding and prevent infection.
Comments: High in calcium and vitamins A, C and K. One of the most widespread medicinal plants, each plant produces up to 20,000 seeds.

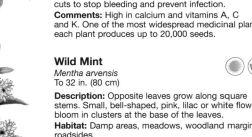

Wild Mint
Mentha arvensis
To 32 in. (80 cm)

Description: Opposite leaves grow along square stems. Small, bell-shaped, pink, lilac or white flowers bloom in clusters at the base of the leaves.
Habitat: Damp areas, meadows, woodland margins, roadsides.
Harvest: Leaves.
Uses: Diuretic, sedative. Tea also treats stomachaches, congestion and sore throats.
Comments: Mint oil is an effective insecticide for killing wasps, ants and cockroaches. Crushed leaves have a mild anesthetic effect and can be rubbed on temples to relieve headaches.

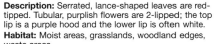

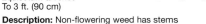

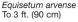

Heal-all
Prunella vulgaris
To 12 in. (30 cm)

Description: Serrated, lance-shaped leaves are red-tipped. Tubular, purplish flowers are 2-lipped; the top lip is a purple hood and the lower lip is often white.
Habitat: Moist areas, grasslands, woodland edges, waste areas.
Harvest: Entire plant.
Uses: Medicinal tea of leaves provides relief from many ailments including sore throat, fevers, gum infections, diarrhea and is believed to heal weaknesses in the liver and heart and respiratory infections. Poultices help wounds to heal.
Comments: The Chinese believed the plant could alter the course of chronic diseases.

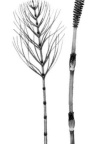

Horsetail
Equisetum arvense
To 3 ft. (90 cm)

Description: Non-flowering weed has stems composed of jointed segments growing in whorls. Fruit is a brownish spore cone.
Habitat: Damp areas, fields, meadows, woodlands, roadsides.
Harvest: Entire plant.
Uses: Diuretic, astringent, stops bleeding and promotes wounds healing. Teas and poultices of the plant are used to treat other problems including skin disorders, kidney problems, joint pain and gout.
Comments: Plant is rich in potassium and calcium.

Aches & Pains – Apply poultice of plantain, chickweed, or wild garlic.

Allergies – Nettle (2-3 cups of tea a day will reduce itching and sneezing).

Bleeding & Cuts – Make poultice of plantain, yarrow leaves or horsetail to stop bleeding.

Clean Wounds, Heal Sores – Use expressed juice of the leaves of wild onion, wild garlic or chickweed. Make a decoction of white oak bark or burdock root. Pine sap helps draw splinters out.

Colds & Sore Throats – Make decoction of willow bark or plantain leaves. Drink tea made of mint leaves, burdock roots, mallow or mullein flowers or roots. Gargle decoction of mint leaves to relieve sore throat.

Constipation – Decoction of dandelion leaves, walnut bark or rose hips.

Cramps – Tea of mullein or yarrow leaves and flowers.

Decongestant – Tea of mullein or mint leaves.

Diarrhea – Drink tea of raspberry, blackberry or cinquefoil roots or a decoction of white oak bark. Use with caution. You can also stop diarrhea by eating campfire ashes or white clay.

Fungus – Treat with decoction of walnut leaves or oak bark. Apply often and expose affected area to sunlight.

Headache – Willow bark (chewed raw, as a tea or decoction), mint (rub oil from leaves on temples).

Hemorrhoids – Treat externally with oak bark tea or expressed juice of plantain leaves.

Itching, Insect Bites & Sunburn – Crush jewelweed stems and apply juice to affected area. Apply poultice of jewelweed to sunburns.

Tooth & Gum Care – Use cattail shoots as toothbrush.

PLANTS SORTED BY EFFECT

Astringent – Draws tissues together, dries up secretions – plantain, yarrow, mullein, raspberry, white oak, cinquefoil, walnut, black willow, yellowroot, horsetail.

Diuretic – Increases urine flow – horsetail, sheep sorrel, dandelion, sassafras, pitch pine, black willow, yarrow, mullein, wild garlic, plantain, wild mint.

Expectorant – Promotes expulsion of phlegm, relieving coughs – plantain, wild garlic, mullein.

Inflammation Reduction – Reduces inflammation and irritation, absorbs moisture and toxins, helps wounds heal – plantain, mullein, yarrow, jewelweed, black walnut, white oak, white pine, pitch pine, black willow, yellowroot, cattail, heal-all, horsetail.

Fever Reduction – Boneset, sheep sorrel, willow, sassafras, tulip poplar, yarrow, heal-all.

Sedative – Slows body functions and promotes relaxation – tea of mint or nettle leaves.

Tonic – Strengthens and restores vitality – nettle, dandelion, yarrow, boneset, black willow, white oak, black walnut, dwarf cinquefoil.